Girl

get off the

couch

**Stop the self-hate and
lose the weight**

DR. RADISHA BROWN

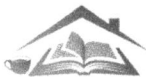

JESUS, COFFEE, & PRAYER

info@drradisha.com – Author Dr. Radisha Brown
www.jesuscoffeeandprayer@gmail.com – Publishing House

ISBN: 978-0-9998188-4-8 (Paperback)

ISBN: 978-0-9998188-5-5 (eBook)

Publisher:
Jesus, Coffee, and Prayer Christian Publishing House
P.O box 691204
Charlotte, NC 28227

www.jesuscoffeeandprayer.com

Chief Editor: Angel Fairley

Cover/Layout/Design: Eswari Kamireddy

Foreword by: Kim HoneyCutt

Photographers: Crystale the Funtographer &
Melissa Heemer

Dedication

I would like to dedicate this book to all the amazing
women that have touched my life. You believed in me
when I did not believe in myself. You helped me
dream beyond what I thought possible. You encouraged and loved me through many roadblocks, setbacks, and obstacles. I stand for every woman that
has ever felt alone, unloved, hopeless, and ashamed. I
am my sister's keeper.

In Loving Memory

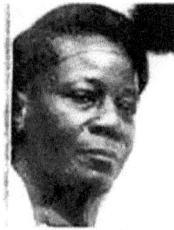

To my grandmother, **Bessie Mae Freeman:** You are the most *amazing* woman that I have ever met. Your life lessons helped me to find the light during my darkest moments. If God allows me to be only 10% of the woman you were- while here on earth, then I would be considered *blessed*. Your constant prayers have protected me on my journey. **You will always be my** *SHERO*!

Table of Contents

Foreword

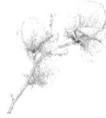

From the first chapter of *Girl, Get off the Couch* I felt connected to Dr. Radisha Brown's trauma and could already detect her resiliency. She does an excellent job of capturing the reader's attention and provoking an appetite for more of her psychological knowledge. This is an excellent read for anyone who is seeking motivation to awaken their personal internal passion for a renewed life.

Kim Honeycutt, MSW, LCSW, CCFC, LCAS
Author of *But Your Mother Loves You*
Psychotherapist & President of icuTalks mental health ministry

Endorsement

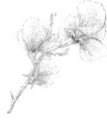

"Dr. Radisha Brown cultivated the strength she needed to kick her food addiction to the curb and lose 80lbs. She now empowers other women to do the same. With simple-not easy-yet effective tips, women are encouraged to take the necessary changes to be successful~ no matter the goal. Girl, Get Off the Couch is the perfect combination of honesty and inspiration that makes for a great read! Whether you just want to be more aware of what you're eating, lose 5lbs or 100, Dr. Radisha's journey inspires all of us to *get off the couch!*"

Bethany Smith, E-RYT
www.bethanysmithyoga.com
@bethanysmithyoga
Nationally recognized Yoga Teacher

Acknowledgments

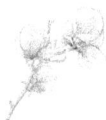

First and foremost, I would like to thank God Almighty for giving me the courage, strength and passion to write this book. Jesus you have given me the power to believe in my passion and pursue my dreams. I could never have done this without the faith I have in you, the Almighty.

My sister, **Stephanie Cruz**: I can barely find the words to express all the wisdom, love and support you have given me all my life. You are my #1 fan and for that I am eternally grateful.

My dad, **Bernard Wright**: Thank you for your unwavering belief in me~ even when I doubted myself. You are not only my dad but also my friend, mentor and coach. I am blessed to call you dad.

My foster parents: **Karen and Alan Morton**: Thank you for giving me a home and encouraging me to get an education. Without your guidance and support I would not be here today. You changed my life.

My sisters: **Alberta, Almeta, Crystal, Cosandra, Symfoni, Tekesha, Yasmin, Karisma** thank you for loving me. I can always count on your support and that means so much. I also know that you would gang up on anybody that comes for me. (laughs) I love you so much!

My brothers: **Kasiem, Jamel, Sheik, Devine, Brian, Brandon**: Thank you for your protection and support. Your faith in me has helped me endure difficult times; I love you more than words could express.

Reginald Kitchens: Thank you for encouraging me to continue this journey on days that I wanted to give up. Thank for supporting my dreams and never doubting my path. I will always be grateful for your love and support.

Dionne Dunn: You helped me to start this book journey. You encouraged me to be vulnerable so that I could help people. Thank you for your guidance and support.

Nicole Pauling: You started as my intern and have grown to be one of my closest friends. You have been a gift from God and I am eternally grateful for your support.

MC Walker: Thank you for believing in this book and helping me to put it down in writing. Your guidance helped me to finally complete this 2 year book journey.

Minister Nakita Davis: Thank you for your passion and support. You have made my dreams come true with the publication of my baby. I will always be grateful! You are one of my biggest fans and I thank God for you!

Kim Honeycutt: Thank you for supporting me on this journey. Your words have touched my heart in an amazing way. May God continue to light your path as you help others to heal.

Bethany Smith: Since the day we met we have been kindred spirits. We share stories of struggle but a tremendous love of Jesus. Thank you for all of your advice. I am so grateful that we met.

Family, Friends and Neighbors: Thank you so very much for believing in me. There have been so many times when I wanted to give up but your words of encouragement gave me courage to continue. You will never understand how much that support changed my life. I am forever grateful.

Facebook Friends: Thank you for sharing and liking my page. Some of you have shown me so much love and support. I am truly grateful! I always say "there is nothing like a good Facebook friend!"

**Special Thanks to My Launch Team-
Your Support was invaluable!**

Almeta Brown

Dionne Dunn

Toya Y. Moore

Kissha Myers

Dorothy Samuel

Monica Williams

Introduction

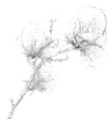

Bessie Mae Freeman, my grandmother, was the greatest woman that I ever met in life. She raised me and my four siblings because my mother, Loretta, was a teenaged parent. Loretta had her first kid at the age of 16, my oldest sister Stephanie; then I came two years later, my sister Cassina came two years after that, then my brother Kasiem, and one year after him my youngest brother Jamel. My mother was busy, to say the least; or as the elderly would say, she was fast in them streets. My mother was pretty much nonexistent in our lives; we would see her from time to time, but she'd just float in and out. She was more of a friend than a parent. My grandmother would always say that my mother was a restless soul and needed to chase the wind. The only thing I wanted in the world was to be loved. It didn't really matter to me how that love showed up in my life. I just needed to know that it existed in my world.

My mother brought five children into the world and left her mark on the inside. She would say to us, "I left y'all with momma. I knew she would take care of y'all because I can't. That was probably the truest statement she ever made in her life. My mother battled alcohol and drugs for as long as I can remember; my grandmother, Bessie, was our saving grace.

This is not your ordinary tale of food addiction or a typical weight loss journey. It's a poetic and poignant love affair with food. Food became a remedy to understanding myself, exploring the world, solving problems, and learning to overcome the harsh realities of my upbringing.

Why now? Why write this book at this chapter in my life? Truth be told, I've been writing this book for as far back as I can remember. Something led me to pick up a pen and paper and begin to write instead of just drowning my tears in my pillow. Write to explain the reasons my waist was constantly expanding before my eyes; write to explain my frequent need to bake things in the middle of the night because of my sweet tooth. I have battled with my weight for a great portion of my life. When it came down to looking at everything within me to understand myself, food was the connection. No, I didn't break up with food or turn my back on all the things I love to eat. Instead I learned to channel that energy into other places and create a life of balance.

My grandmother Bessie stored inside of me all the things I would need along my walk as a woman. She taught me that a woman was more than just a birthing machine or an object of pleasure for the opposite sex. She taught me to love myself and value the woman I am becoming. Although she taught me everything she loved and knew in her years, she always added a little food for the special occasion. That's when I realized within myself that food and I were enemies – that someday food would ultimately control my life.

If you picked up this book and assumed that it was just another book about why you can't fit inside your jeans, or why your boyfriend keeps telling you your butt's getting big – then this is not the book for you. Yep! This is for the woman who is ready and willing to do the internal work to discover her self-worth in life. This book is for the young woman who is searching for answers and solutions to having a healthy and positive relationship with food. This book is for someone who needs to know that her weight loss journey needs to be documented to encourage others to take the first step.

1

Sugar is the Devil

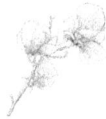

Every major life transformation begins with making the choice to change. That means you must take things into your own hands and decide that it's time to do things differently. When it comes to weight loss, that means you must decide whether or not you're going to let what you eat control you, or if you're going to control what you eat.

The first thing you need to realize when changing your diet is that sugar has to go. I know that sounds tough because it seems like sugar is in almost everything (under the guise of fructose), but you simply won't be able to transform your life in the way you want if you decide you're too weak to fight off the evil force of sugar. Remember that weakness is a state of mind you choose, not one that is inherent to you as a person. Sugar is the devil; and it's waiting around every corner to suck you in and divert you from your path to glory. You can't let that happen, and more importantly, you should know that you have the power to ensure that it doesn't.

Sugar was going to kill me. My doctor told me that I was on my way to developing type II diabetes. That's when I knew I had to make a change and rid my life of sugar. This wasn't just a matter of feeling good about myself; it was a matter of life and death. I made the choice to live and my first step to making that choice was realizing that my life depended on making a change.

For me, cutting sugar out of my diet meant pouring sweet tea down the drain. I can't even begin to describe how hard it was. Sweet tea was such a staple of my diet — so much so that I was probably drinking forty to fifty ounces of sweet tea a day. And I'm from the south, so that means the recipe is basically sugar with tea added; not the other way around. You should know that I ate fried chicken every day. And my beverage of choice to wash down that fried chicken? Sweet tea. I thought that the combination of fried chicken and sweet tea was helping to ease the pain I felt from my sense of worthlessness, but I soon learned that sugar only increased my feelings of despair.

You may not know it, but sugar actually intensifies feelings of depression and anxiety. If you're already struggling with depression then sugar is only going to bring you down further. If you aren't struggling with depression, a diet that's heavily sugar based can make you vulnerable to suffering. I ate all that fried chicken and consumed all that sugar and drank all that sweet tea because I didn't feel good about who I was as a person; sugar was only making it worse. It probably goes without saying, but sugar destroys your body in addition to negatively affecting your mindset. Heavy sugar intake can cause you to look older because sugar causes wrinkles by interfering with the way your body breaks down protein fibers like collagen. So, not only did I feel bad about myself on the inside but on the outside as well.

The fact that I didn't like the way I looked or felt, coupled with the fact that my doctor said my diet was my sentence to death row, made me realize I had to eliminate as much sugar as I could from my diet; that meant no more sweet tea. I made the choice to go from sweet tea to water. It seems like a simple decision, but following through wasn't as easy as I thought it would be. I learned that there is such a thing as sugar withdrawal. My body and my mind were craving sugar like crazy. I was nauseous. I had headaches. I didn't understand what was going on. But once I found out how addictive sugar is, it started to make sense.

It turns out that sugar is eight times more addictive than cocaine. I couldn't believe it! No wonder it was so hard to kick my sweet tea habit. At first, I was ashamed of my cravings. I thought they were my fault and that something was wrong with me. But when I realized it was an addiction, I knew that I no longer needed to feel shame. No one should feel ashamed of any addiction — whether it's drugs, alcohol, sex, or food. Addiction is a medical issue and it can drive the choices that you make. Once you realize you're an addict, you can become empowered to make the decision to change your life. It was clear to me that I was addicted to food — to sugar. I had to take a stand and tell myself I would no longer succumb to my food addiction.

2

The Word No is Anointed

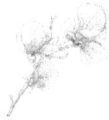

You have to remember that during your weight loss journey you're going to be confronted with temptation. I've already mentioned that you can be addicted to food just like you can be addicted to drugs or alcohol, and even sex. With any and every addiction comes temptation – it's just the nature of the beast.

When we're tempted with anything, we have to keep in mind one simple, sacred word: NO. The word no is anointed; it's the sacred word that's going to help you fight against cravings and temptations. Remember the old adage just say no to drugs? In this case, it's going to be say no to sugar or say no to fatty foods. Whatever force is bringing you down, whether that be the temptation to eat the foods that are road-blocks on your weight loss journey or the negative emotions that make you want to eat those unhealthy foods, you have to remember to just say no.

"No, I will not let sugar control me. No, I will not give into temptation and eat all that fried food. No, I will not let any negative thinking bring me down today."

Not only do you have to say no to temptations and negative thinking, but there's also going to be times when you might have to say no to the toxic people in your life. That means you can't let people bring you down and make you feel bad about your-self. We already know that a huge part of food addic-tion has to do with how you feel about yourself on the inside. Often, it's the people in our lives that can affect our emotions the most. If there's someone in your life who upsets you and makes you want to turn to food to feel better, you should ask yourself the question, "Do I want this person in my life right now while I'm trying to get better and heal?" Again, the answer is "No."

"No, I do not have time for this person. I can't let this person take up real estate in my head and get in the way of what I'm trying to accomplish."

I said "NO" to my toxic marriage. I know that my ex-husband was a toxic force in my life that caused my feelings of worthlessness to skyrocket; so much so that I felt the only way to cope was to over-eat — further perpetuating the cycle of emotional pain. I was married for ten years. I invested so much of my heart and soul into my marriage, but my husband's actions eventually led to the realization that the marriage I tried so hard to make work was dysfunctional and ultimately destroying my mind, body, and soul.

You see, my ex was a serial cheater. It was his actions that brought feelings of torture and turmoil that I found to be absolutely unbearable; my whole world, including my views on love and the holy sanctity of marriage, had been turned completely upside down. A man that I loved with so much passion couldn't love me for me. He had to find his love elsewhere with other women. How was I supposed to take such heartbreak? I was hurt and confused, and sought to do everything within my power to change the situation — mainly by trying to change him. Even after finding out about my husband's infidelity, I did my best to make it work.

The tipping point that made me realize I had to do something different was when I found out about the second time he cheated on me. I had this intuition in my gut that he'd been fooling around on me again but I didn't want to accept it or even confront it. I was terrified to have the conversation because I didn't know what the confrontation would bring. Would my marriage end in ruins? I debated for weeks whether or not I should talk to him about it. I didn't know if confronting it would do any good. Even if I knew, even he admitted it, what would be next?

I eventually mustered up the strength and courage to ask my ex-husband what was going on. At first, he lied, but something still didn't seem right. He later admitted the truth, but did so in a way that didn't seem to make any sense. He told me he was "raped". He tried to put the blame on someone else instead of taking responsibility for his infidelity. I couldn't believe that a man I cared for so much didn't even have the decency and respect for me to tell me straight up and honestly what he had been up to. It made me feel as if there was something wrong with me, as if it was all my fault; like it was me who put him in the position where he felt he was forced to lie and deceive me.

We went to counseling. We even renewed our vows. I thought that the help of others could save our marriage, but I ultimately understood that I had to take control of the situation. The way I took control was by saying NO. I had to tell both myself and my husband that I would no longer put up with being treated as if I didn't matter. I would no longer take the psychological abuse of feeling neglected by someone whom I deeply and passionately loved. Taking control of the situation meant letting go. It meant understanding that controlling my ex-husband's actions was an impossibility. It meant saying to my husband that I could no longer take his infidelities and lies. I had to look deep within myself and ask myself whether or not I was willing to put up with such cruelty and deception. I had to ask myself whether or not I deserved the treatment my ex-husband so unjustly gave me. I said NO.

I knew I couldn't change my husband. When I asked myself whether I could change him, and firmly answered with a no, that's when I was able to make the real changes I needed. I couldn't waste time trying to change him; I had to make the change within myself to become stronger by refusing to accept his infidelity. When I realized I couldn't change him and that I had to change myself, I was absolutely terrified. Even though he hurt me, cut my chest wide open and left my wounded heart on the ground, I still loved him. Yes, despite what he did to me, I still loved him.

But would I take the suffering any longer? No, I would not. I had to reject the love I felt and learn how to let that love go. I had to learn how to say no to a man I loved and to a feeling I so badly wanted to hold on to.

You have to say no to toxicity or you aren't going to get better. My relationship was toxic because despite all of my husband's despicable behavior, it was so hard to let my love for him die. The same goes with my love affair with food. I loved to eat in the way that was killing me, or at least I thought I did. I had to say no to the love I felt for my husband and I had to say no to the love I felt for the foods I knew would cause my demise.

In this particular case, the word no is an affirmation of sorts. When you say no to what makes you suffer, you're affirming your self-worth, greatness, and strength. Realizing that saying no is a clear sign of your strength is key. It's hard to say no. Sometimes it's the hardest word to say. Doing what is hardest to do takes a tremendous amount of courage and strength. In this case, you need to have the courage and strength to say no. When you do so, it's going to exponentially increase your confidence and help you achieve your goal. And that goal is being the best person that you can be – being the best version of you. Weight loss is just a means of becoming the confident and beautiful human being that you already are. I guarantee you that saying no to temptation, negative thinking, and toxic people will give you the confidence you need to lose weight and reach the ultimate goal: self-love and self-worth.

3

Visualize the Change

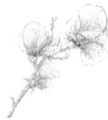

To make a major life change, you'll first have to visualize it. That means really getting the clearest mental picture of what that change is going to look like. You need the most detailed picture possible in order to achieve your goal, otherwise you won't really understand what the goal is. For me, losing weight was more than just changing my physical appearance; it was about changing the way I felt about myself. Weight loss is all about becoming a new you. When you decide to take the steps towards becoming a new you, you have to ask yourself, "What is a new

me going to look like? Who exactly am I going to become and what do I do to make that transformation?"

Visualizing the change means visualizing both
the goal and the tough road it takes to achieve that
goal. You have to think about and understand what
your journey is going to look like every step of the
way. I had to take a strong look at myself and a strong
look at the person I wanted to be in order to reach a
sense of self-love and balance. It was a new inner and
spiritual self that I had to visualize. I had to do more
than just get a good picture of what it would be like
to change my eating habits. When you look inward
and visualize who you want to become, it means visualizing how you're going to live your life. That means
more than envisioning yourself saying that you're a
confident, strong, unique individual who loves her-
self. Ask what the life of that strong, confident, and
unique person you wish to become looks like – what
that person does day in and day out. Visualize the
roles that confidence and strength and love play in
your life.

There are so many questions you can ask yourself
when you reflect upon what a new you will look like.
What will my work life look like? What will my routines look like? What will my relationships look like?
How am I going to treat people? How am I going to
treat myself? When you're trying to answer these

questions, remember that you're basically assessing your future perspective and attitude. You're putting into question your current attitudes and making a conscious effort to see how your thought process can transform over time, and how that transformation is going to affect every aspect of your life.

Losing weight means cultivating a new lifestyle. Lifestyles begin with a set of beliefs and attitudes that translate to how you live every moment of every day. If you make no effort to understand how every slight attitude adjustment you make plays a part in the way you live, then you probably won't reach and realize your full potential. You won't be able to thrive, grow, love, and live in the way you deserve. Think for a second about all the changes you're going to make when you reach the decision to lose weight. If you haven't already figured it out, you should know that the changes are so much more than a new diet with some exercise thrown in. At least for me, it was so much more. And if you're reading this book, then the same probably goes for you. I ate the way I did because I felt alone, depressed, unloved, unworthy, and like I was never enough. When I ate to try to alleviate the pain, it only made the pain worse. I felt caught in an endless and vicious cycle that left me feeling nothing close to full. I felt completely empty inside, and that's what needed to change. Yes, I wanted to change my waist size but what I really needed to do was change the way I viewed myself and the way my views affected how I lived, loved, worked, and played – none of which I felt I was doing in the way I knew I should and could be able to do.

If you don't think about how a change in perspective is going to affect the way you live, then you won't know what changes to make. You have to understand how your thoughts of self-loathing play a part in every aspect of what you do. Once you gain a deep understanding of how your attitude affects everything from your interpersonal relationships to your work life, then you'll be able to develop the plan you need to feel empowered. This is about so much more than weight loss. You are examining the relationship between your inner-self and food, visualizing the relationship between feelings and actions; and really, overeating is just a small part among the many aspects of your life that needs to change.

4

Perfect is the Enemy of Good

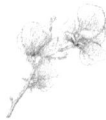

Nobody is perfect regardless of who they are. You probably already know that. And hopefully you know that your weight loss journey isn't going to go perfectly, nor should you make perfection your end goal. Even once you lose weight, you aren't going to hit some fixed point of perfection. You have to remember here that losing the weight and maintaining the mindset that helped you lose the weight to begin with are two separate processes.

The key word here is process, and processes are always in constant flux. You're going to have your ups and down when losing the weight, and you're going to have your ups and downs when it comes to keeping your negative thoughts in check. I'm not saying you shouldn't strive to be the best you can be. What you should know, though, is that being the best you can be means that you understand everything isn't going to go exactly as you plan. Not only does being the best mean you understand this, but it also means you can accept it. If you can accept that the process isn't always going to be perfect, then you're doing a good job. Perfect is the enemy of good. If you expect everything to be perfect all the time, you're never going to lose the desired amount of weight, and more importantly you're never going to be able to keep a positive mindset which will ensure that you keep the weight off.

Remember, it's a change in attitude and perspective that's going to help you lose weight. A huge part of having the right attitude means learning to roll with the punches if something gets in your way and derails the perfection you aim to achieve. When I said earlier that you have to visualize the change, part of that means you have to visualize how you're going to deal with bumps in the road. Once you lose weight, you'll still have to work every day to make sure you don't fall into the trap of negative thoughts.

Even though I lost the weight I needed to lose so I could feel good about myself, I still have to put in the emotional work every day that helped me get to where I am. And you know what? I'm going to have to do it tomorrow, and the next day, and the next day after that. Working on yourself never ends, and that's more than ok. You never want to stop working on yourself. When you constantly strive for more, that doesn't mean you aren't good enough; it means you're putting in the work you need to succeed.

The problem with the perception of perfection is that it's a standard that no one meets because that standard doesn't exist. Despite that, we all try to meet that standard. That means so many people out there are trying to find and maintain some state that is unachievable; not because no one has the strength to try, but because you can't achieve what isn't real. There is no such thing as perfection, and if you imagine that your weight loss path will be perfect, then your path will be filled with countless roadblocks and detours. The attempt to meet the standard of perfection is only going to set you back. You already know that overeating is simply a way to cope when you feel unbearably low. If your journey doesn't align with some crazy idea of perfection (which it won't), don't set yourself up for a mountain of negative thinking that can feel almost impossible to climb. When something feels impossible, it becomes so easy to give up. Giving up is the last thing you want to do.

You're bound to encounter stress and frustration on your way to changing your mindset and shedding those pounds. Attempts at perfect will do nothing more than exacerbate that stress and frustration, and you'll turn to food to cope. What we're changing here is coping mechanisms, and an attempt at perfection won't give you the slightest chance at change. For so many of us, the idea of perfection is what makes us suffer to begin with. We feel all that unworthiness and loneliness because we try to be perfect. You've got to remember that if you try to be perfect, you'll never feel like you're enough.

Never feeling like I was enough was a huge reason that I ate to the point of self-destruction, nearly killing myself. I ate that way because I couldn't reach unrealistic expectations, and that only caused me to eat more. If you want to break the cycle you have to forget about perfection and just focus on the process. When the emphasis of your efforts is making changes every day, you're going to get the results you want. Again, that point is simply reaching a place where you realize that working on your inner-self is something that needs to be done every day and that it is a perpetual process.

Comparing My Own Success to the Standard of Perfection

Even once I began to get my diet on track, I still had my handful of setbacks; the main one being my love of bread. Once I learned about the negative effects of gluten, I knew I had to cut bread from my diet. Cutting it out wasn't easy in the least. The fact that I even had to make another dietary change was disheartening. Even though I understand that maintaining spiritual balance and a healthy weight is a process, it didn't exactly occur to me that that meant continually trying out new things in my diet.

So, I cut out the bread, but I craved it like crazy. Just like sugar and fried foods, bread was a huge staple of my diet − even after I took steps in the right direction. Not only did I desire bread throughout the day, but that desire even permeated my sleep. I kept have this recurring dream of myself sitting at a table, with a smorgasbord of breads − cornbread, yeast rolls, all hot and buttery and sweet and ready for me to eat. I'd wake up and couldn't believe it. I thought I had reached success; why was I still craving what was killing me? Just having the cravings made me feel like I was doing it all wrong. I thought my love affair with food was over, and when still had to fight off cravings for bread, it made me feel like I was a failure. My cravings became so intense that sometimes I would drive to restaurants that served yeast rolls and indulge. This would happen even after I already ate a healthy meal. I was doing so well yet I would negate my progress by giving in to my strong desires to stuff myself with bread. It was as if my whole journey towards transformation had been a total waste of time, effort, and energy. But what I really needed to understand in order to get to a better place was that my setback really wasn't a setback at all; it was part of the process towards betterment.

My success wasn't perfect. So what? I had to realize that nobody's success, no matter who they are, is perfect. As I've already said, the closest you can get to perfection is accepting that behavioral and spiritual change is a continual process. Perfection is a process; not a destination. And setbacks are just an inevitable part of that process. Anyone who's ever had success experienced setbacks along the way; it just comes with the territory. Understand that roadblocks show up throughout your journey, causing you to take many a detour. The road to success is circuitous. You're not just going to go from point A to point B. The best thing that you can do is expect and accept that setbacks will happen so that you'll be prepared when you're up against any obstacle you face.

Being prepared means having a plan in place. Tons of journaling prompts are all about creating a plan to overcome roadblocks that could potentially (not definitely) sabotage your efforts to a healthy mind, body, and spirit. What you have to do when journaling is create roadblock solutions so that you won't be caught totally off guard when you hit a wall. Think about a situation like a big office party or holiday party and make a plan for what you might do when you're confronted with a buffet of sweets. If you already have a plan in place to fight off any triggers, you'll know what to do when you see that spread.

You're also going to want to be prepared when doing grocery shopping. That might sound a little odd seeing as how grocery shopping isn't a scenario or situation per se, but grocery stores are indeed filled with food, and that includes the food you know are detrimental to your progress. That's why you should make a shopping list. Be prepared for what you're going to get before you get there, that way you aren't overwhelmed by all the options or caught by surprise when you see something you might usually crave. If you know what you want before you show up, if you're prepared, then avoiding unhealthy foods will be easier. You'll know beforehand what aisles to go down and which aisles to steer clear of. It'll help keep unhealthy foods that perpetuate negative thinking out of sight and out of mind. And it's imperative that you don't shop while you're hungry. If you go to the grocery store on an empty stomach, you might very well buy anything that looks the least bit appetizing simply because you feel like you'd eat anything at that point. Instead of just getting what you need at the grocery store, you're just going to end up getting what you want on a whim. Success and preparation go hand in hand, meaning there's no room for compulsive eating.

You have to be regimented. It may sound a little too restrictive, but if you want to lose weight you have to set some guidelines and show a little discipline. If you're hungry at the grocery store — and even worse, without a list — you're going to give in to your cravings and showing restraint is going to be difficult. It's not that you're weak; far from it. It's just that discipline and restraint are inherent in strength. Having strength means that you can have control over your actions, and preparation is key to control. If you find yourself struggling with control, though, don't beat yourself up about it. Perfection is by no means synonymous with control. For our purposes, in terms of perfection and control, just think of perfection as a state of mind where you understand that control leads to success. If you lose control for a moment, it doesn't mean you aren't perfect. It's all part of the process; you have to remember that.

Let's not forget that preparation is all about having the right tools — the right weapons to fight off setbacks. In this case, that means you should always be prepared with healthy foods in your arsenal. Let's say you're at work and you get hungry during the middle of the day and are craving a snack. Instead of heading over to the vending machine and getting something like chips or a candy bar, you should bring low-calorie and heart-healthy foods with you. Try fruit or vegetables like cucumbers. Nuts, trail mix, and hummus are also great go-to healthy snacks.

And if you can't seem to control cravings, remember you can always turn to water. Drinking a nice, tall glass of water can trick your body into thinking it's full.

Don't get discouraged if you find yourself struggling even once you've lost the weight that is bringing you down. It doesn't mean you're a failure. When I noticed that I still wanted to turn to food in order to cope even though I had reached my goal, I felt like a fraud — like I never really reached success. I thought success and perfection meant ridding myself of cravings entirely, but it just doesn't work that way. If you're of the mindset that every time you have a craving for unhealthy foods that you're a failure, then you're only setting yourself up to return to negative coping mechanisms. Think about it: if you crave unhealthy food and feel like you've failed because you have that craving, you're bound to get depressed and turn to food to make you feel better, which we already know is making you unhappy to begin with. The cycle is vicious, but being mindful of that cycle and how you can fall into it is going to help you keep a positive attitude.

I've said it so many times and I can't say it enough. Perfection is a process and not an end point. The journey never ends and understanding that is the only way you're going to be able to maintain the success you want. Yes, you're going to have setbacks. But setbacks are part of the road to achieving your goals. Success means you can overcome. If there's no roadblocks, then really, what have you overcome? Be prepared to struggle with your notions of perfection; it's only going to make you stronger in the end.

5

Food Affects Your Mood

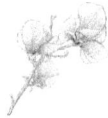

The food we eat and the way we eat it can either make or break the connection between our mind, body, and spirit. When we use food as a way to cope with the troubles that cripple us, the strength of the links in the chain of mind, body, and spirit only weaken. We think overeating can help us heal, but instead it hurts us. Overeating gets so complicated because of the emotional feedback loop it creates. We overeat because we suffer, and yet we suffer because we overeat. This is the case with all negative coping mechanisms just like drugs, alcohol, or hypersexuality. Knowing how addiction magnifies the depression we feel, food was an addiction I had to break.

Think for a moment about the cycle of my food addiction. I felt unloved and worthless. I turned to food as a way to ease my pain; but it only multiplied my misery tenfold. When I looked at myself in the mirror, I hated the way that I looked and felt. I hated myself more than ever knowing that I was headed down the road to death at full throttle. Not only did overeating intensify my depression and my emotional need to overeat, but the specific food I ate intensified it as well.

Remember all the sweet tea I drank? Remember how I learned I had a physical addiction to sugar? I was hooked on both a physical and emotional level, causing breakage in the bond of my mind, body, and spirit. My brain chemicals were being toyed with by sugar. My body was blowing up. My spirit was crushed. My mindset was filled with self-loathing and the lack of love in my life. I wanted to love myself but my food addiction put love so far out of reach.

Food affects your mood. So often we overlook the way that nutrition shapes our road to wellness and wholeness. Nutrition is integral to the mastery of emotional balance. If we don't take care of our bod-ies, our mindset suffers. If you want to find self-worth, you have to care for yourself as if you're worth it (of course, you know you are). Our mental health and physical health are intertwined in more ways than we think. It's all about the way you treat yourself. If you destroy your body by overeating — if you treat your body poorly and without respect — self-respect and self-love on emotional level is impossible to achieve.

How can you love something you don't respect? When we think about the link between the respect we have for our bodies and the respect we have for ourselves, it's no wonder overeating causes so much despair. In order to thrive, it's so important that we love ourselves; and you simply can't love yourself if you don't treat yourself with the respect and care you deserve.

Overeating was stripping my sense of autonomy and control. I ate to comfort myself and escape the feelings of weakness that crushed my spirit. I felt weak. I had to understand, though, that I was not weak; I was simply in the grips of a food addiction that was killing me. One of the first steps to weight loss is understanding that you have more control over the situation than you think. Overeating is not a weakness. You only feel weak; you can't recognize the strength you hold within. If you just take a close look at yourself, and see how beautiful and strong you really are, you'll understand that empowerment is more than possible.

Don't let food affect your mood. You have the strength to control how you look at yourself and the world. It's up to you and not your addiction. All you have to do is take small steps toward eating in a way that won't cloud your thinking. Those feelings of self-love will come to you; and you can welcome them with open arms.

6

Everything Looks Good on Paper

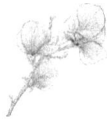

Getting some pen and paper and outlining a road map of your weight loss journey is an excellent way to know what you're up against. Putting your goals down on paper will help you better visualize the changes you want to make. But you have to keep in mind something we've already talked about − the poison of perfection.

When you see all the steps you want to take written out neatly on paper, it's going to seem perfect. But, there's always a chance that you might deviate from your plan, or you might decide that plan doesn't quite fit your specific needs. Everything looks good on paper; but that doesn't mean it necessarily is good or that it's going to go as smoothly as an outline might make it seem.

Yes, of course, you want a plan. But doing your best to stick to it can be tough. Staying on course is a challenge, for sure, but you have to be ready to face that challenge; you can't give up if everything doesn't work out exactly as you planned. You also have to understand that just because everything is written out nice and neat doesn't mean the journey's going to be easy. I don't say this to discourage you, but to prepare you. When you see your journey mapped out you might think, "That's it? That's all I have to do? Just check this stuff off the list and everything will go fine?" Yes, you'll know what you have to do. But just because you know what to do doesn't mean you won't be presented with hard times along the way. An outline is certainly meant to make things easier, but it's not going to automatically make the process easy. The same goes for this book. It's here for you to turn to when needed – to inspire you, motivate you, comfort you, and offer reassurance. But even though I'm giving you tips I know will guide you to success, I'm not promising you that the process will be a breeze.

The tools you need to equip yourself with and the goals you want to reach seem simple only on the surface. That doesn't mean you lack the strength to follow through with anything you set your mind to, but you should know that following through isn't easy. We all know how much we want to give in sometimes. But one thing I'm challenging you to do is cultivate a mindset that doesn't give in to giving up. Don't allow yourself to get discouraged. It's so easy to put onto paper, but it isn't easy to put into practice. Having a plan is only half the battle; the other half is executing your plan, and having the strength to try to travel the path even if you reach an unexpected fork in the road.

7

Pain Provides Growth

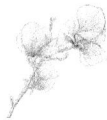

Weight loss is all about developing strength – the strength to change and the strength to persevere. But I'll tell you this: building up strength will always be accompanied by some pain. Pain provides growth. Pain will help you build your strength. It's just like with exercise. Working out and physical activity can often leave you sore. But you know that if you're feeling the pain that you're doing it right. The same goes for your weight loss journey. If you're feeling the pain, you're doing it right.

Again, just because you know the steps to take doesn't mean taking them will be easy. The journey will be painful; it may be scary. Self-examination takes a lot of guts and bravery simply because it is not an easy task. When you look inward, you may find yourself facing some demons you didn't know you had. That can be intimidating and frightening, but we all know the value in confronting our fears. My life has been filled with hardships that at first seemed insurmountable. I grew up in poverty, my parents were absent from my life, and my husband of ten years lied to me and broke my heart. My mother was a drug addict who didn't take care of me and my siblings, my father was out of the picture, and I was raised by my grandmother. After my grandmother passed away, I lived in multiple foster homes. I never knew anything that even came close to stability, and I never even dreamed my accomplishments could be achieved.

People who grew up like me often feel like they don't have a chance at success. It always seemed that people like me just stayed at the bottom while the rest of the world moved all the way up to the top. At first, I didn't understand that I could make something of myself. Why would I think differently? My mother wasted her life, we were always poor, and me and my siblings were considered nothing more than troublemakers. I had nothing and I thought it would stay that way.

Now I have more than I could ever imagine. My foster parents actually encouraged me to go college. They gave me the reassurance I needed so that I could help others and make a difference in people's lives. Even with the reassurance I was given, I wouldn't have been able to believe in myself if I never experienced pain. Once I realized that just getting through my hectic upbringing took great strength, I knew I had the strength to accomplish anything I wanted – and that includes losing weight. But like I already said, strength can only come from pain. You never become stronger if it doesn't hurt along the way.

Pain and My Personal Relationships

The pain caused by my husband's infidelity and deception, which in turn led me to leave him, caused me gut-wrenching pain like I had never felt before. The decision to leave my husband and sever the ties of our love was one of the most difficult decisions of my adult life. Even though my ex-husband hurt me deeply, it was so hard to imagine a life without him. I had been with him for ten years, showing him great love and compassion; and at first, I didn't know how to live a life that was devoid of the love I gave him. To give someone your all, to get nothing back in return, to have the desire to give even when you know that your gift will go unappreciated, to have to take control and stamp out that fiery desire, to let it all go — the pain was practically unbearable.

A life without a love for him seemed unimaginable. Even though I never received back the love and loyalty that I gave, I still didn't know how I was going to go on without him. But the pain I experienced when I ended our relationship, and the initial pain that accompanied my life of loneliness was so integral to my transformation. I've felt so much deep pain, but the disintegration of my marriage gave me the strength to look deep into myself during my time of solitude and change my attitude completely. Of all the pain I've felt that led to my metamorphosis, it's leaving my relationship that contributed most to that change within myself. I have no doubt in my mind that I am who I am — beautiful, strong, and determined — because of the decision to leave my ex-husband.

Without that pain, I never would have decided to open my own business or become a radio show host; without that pain I wouldn't be the person I am today. It's because of my tumultuous relationship and the subsequent heart-crushing pain that I was left with that allowed me to become who I am — it allowed me to be here to listen to you, and to help you move your life in the right direction. I wouldn't be here helping you today if I'd never experienced pain and I probably wouldn't have even wanted to help. It's your pain that makes me want to share my experiences. I want you to know that my upbringing caused pain, that the way I thought about myself caused pain, that my relationship with my husband caused me pain, and that my food addiction caused me pain. Everything in my life that's been a source of pain has made me stronger. If you understand that the same will undoubtedly apply to you, then you'll understand how capable you are of reinventing your mindset and losing weight.

My pain helped me grow into the strong woman I am today, and you should know that you are strong too. But you need to remember that even though I can offer you guidance, it isn't me who is going to give you strength. You are the source of your own strength, and it is your trials and tribulations that allow you to build that strength. Remember that losing weight means learning how to live your life and love yourself differently, and that means learning how to grow. We don't just grow automatically; we need challenges and tough life experience to help us grow. Trust me when I say that growth awaits you. Although it will be painful, that pain will allow you to transform in ways you never thought possible.

8

Working with the Wrong Information Gives You Bad Results

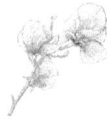

There is a ton of information out there about different diets and approaches to weight loss. Remember, though, that not all information is trustworthy. Working with the wrong information gives you bad results, so you have to make sure you're getting the proper nutritional advice needed to help you live the life you deserve.

While your friends and family members will have advice to offer you, (and hopefully they'll give you their full support), you want to make sure you consult professionals so that you can embark on the best diet for you. Yes, there are definitely general standards that work for everybody; but the extent to which those standards are effective can differ from person to person. If you base your plan off information that is not accurate to your specific nutritional needs, you won't get the results you want. If you don't get the results you want, you might feel that all is hopeless and that you should just give up.

It's so important that you make educated and informed decisions with the help of professionals before you start the weight loss process. Talk to your doctor, find a nutritionist or dietician, and see a therapist or counselor that can help you when the going gets tough. You definitely have it in you to make the changes you need, but you have to be informed in addition to being willing. Don't let misinformation get in the way of the new you.

When the Wrong Information is About Yourself

Let's also remember that wrong information isn't necessarily restricted to the dietary realm. By this I mean that misinformation can also be seen as misbelief; and in our case, specifically misbeliefs about ourselves that others instill in us.

Take my ex-husband, for instance. All of his actions and his attitude led me to believe that I was a worthless human being who was undeserving of the love that we all need. Even after I knew that my husband cheated on me, I still stayed with him because he made me feel like I couldn't do any better. He made me feel like I didn't deserve better. My ex made me believe things about myself that simply are not true. When you hold false beliefs about yourself, how can you expect yourself to succeed in life? The answer is that you can't. You will never tap into your potential as a strong and beautiful human being if you don't believe in yourself. Believing is half the battle; it's the first step you have to take. As I've said countless times, this isn't just about changing the way your body looks; it's about changing the way you think which in turn changes the way you feel. I know that you can achieve anything you want. I believe in you. But do you believe in yourself?

My marriage made it so hard for me to believe in myself, to the point where accomplishing my goals seemed like an insurmountable feat. Even worse, it made it so hard for me to believe in myself because I was scared to want more from life. I almost felt as if I was ungrateful for desiring more than what was handed to me. My husband made me feel absolutely worthless and undeserving; he made me feel as if I were lucky to have what he gave me at all, as if he was doing me a favor by staying with me. I had to believe that it was ok to want more and that I deserved it. If I wasn't able to overcome the way my ex made me feel, then I wouldn't have developed the courage and strength to reach where I am today. If you go into your weight loss journey with the belief that you aren't worth it, then bad results are inevitable. Negative thinking is going to derail you, and you'll never be able to reach your destination.

When it comes to weight loss, holding false beliefs is just as detrimental, and probably even more so, as working with the wrong dietary information. I want you to achieve holistic success; that means having the right tools in place for a healthy body, but most importantly having the tools you need for a healthy mind. You can't neglect your belief system if you want to lose weight. You have to work every day on shaping a belief system that is devoid of negative thinking. Don't let toxic people make you believe things about yourself that aren't true. Misbelief and misinformation are one and the same; you have to remember that if you're going to begin working towards a transformation.

9

Forgiveness is Key

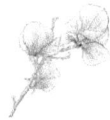

In my formative years, when someone hurt me I would cancel them, as we say today. If I trusted you and you hurt me, I wanted nothing else to do with you. I would carry that pain around inside of me. I would use it as venom against others to keep people from getting too close to me. It wasn't until my adult years that I realized how toxic and destructive this mentality was to me and to others.

The way I lived my whole life was practically centered around certain relationships. While I love my family and the dynamics of each relationship, it caused me to protect myself from others. The people in my family looked to me as a shoulder to lean on in times of frustration, doubt, and even stress. I was there for the people I loved in more ways than one. It was easy to transition this thinking process into the real world. I assumed right off the bat that people would always be good to me because I was good to them. Imagine the depth of my pain and anxiety when I received the short end of the stick in my friendships and relationships. When the person I loved in a platonic or non-platonic relationship broke my heart or disappointed me. I wanted nothing to do with them. I was intent on rebuilding that relationship with someone new. When that didn't work, I took the pain and angst for their actions out on myself. I was the reason this relationship failed. Or I couldn't get past the depth of the pain the other person caused me so I blamed myself for being so trusting and naive. For years, I carried the weight of anger inside of me and released it all into my love affair with food.

Food could never let me down. It was always easy and readily available to satisfy the missing pieces in my life. I'd sit on my couch for hours stuffing my face with fried chicken, doughnuts, ice cream, and any kind of biscuit I could wrap my fingers around. Food was a silent and guilty pleasure. Food comforted my troubles whether I was feeling good, bad, or in between. The problem was that my issues would soon return like rain in August. They were still there wait-ing for me to address them properly. No amount of food could ever take the pain and loneliness I would feel on the inside.

Forgiveness is not about expecting the other per-son to feel guilty or regretful about their actions. For-giveness begins with you having the willpower and understanding to know that people make mistakes. Yet, you have the ability to look past their errors and give them a second chance to correct them. The hardest part for me was learning how to look inward and forgive those in my life who had done me wrong. My mother was not in my life and that left me feeling abandoned. I used to believe that if I prayed hard enough to God that my mother would magically cor-rect her actions. She would somehow become the mother my siblings and I needed. Things didn't work out the way I intended. They worked out for the best the way God planned them. It took quite a bit of time to learn to forgive my mother. It took me becoming a woman and learning the ways of the world. Under-standing that my mother was sick. Sick people need forgiveness just like the rest of us. Forgiving my mother was the breaking of the chain I needed to al-low myself to begin to heal internally. Forgiving oth-ers gave me the permission I needed to see people not as my own perception of who they should be, but for who they truly are.

Forgiveness is freedom and room to grow emotionally and spiritually. When I learned to walk freely in my power, I clothed myself in forgiveness because I needed to learn that I am a continuous work in progress. I make mistakes and I expect someone to forgive me. Although some apologies may never come, I learned to forgive people anyway. I empower myself when I choose to forgive and flow through life as God intended.

10

Morning Ritual for Success

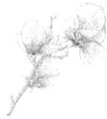

B y now, you're probably thinking that my food affair was limited to my relationship with the couch. After all, the couch was the center of my universe when I would pop open a bag of chips. My couch comforted me through breakups, work deadlines, lonely nights indoors, and abusive friendships. That is, until I became serious about changing my bad habits and adopting a new lifestyle.

Most people believe that if you join the gym and eat a few veggies during the week, your bad habits will disappear on their own. Not quite my friends. My bad habits followed me around like they were my children.

Everywhere I went, I could see remnants of the behavior I created to get my body and mind in poor condition. Coffee mugs everywhere I looked in my home because I used to need that extra boost to get up in the morning. My couch was the truth teller of all the things I enjoyed during my down time. Cookie crumbs, potato chip bags, and candy wrappers often popped up out of nowhere. To make matters worse, my bad habits would start in the morning and run my entire day. I am guilty of loving my rest time in my bed. I enjoy sleeping late and waking up late to cook a good breakfast like my grandma. Before I knew it, two eggs, grits, hash browns, toast, and bacon are on my plate. I'd wash it all down with my coffee and go back to resting on my couch. By mid afternoon, I would feel lethargic and ready to eat again. My poor morning routine went on for years. I knew I needed to make some changes sooner than later. That change needed to begin with my morning routine.

I'd be fibbing if I told you I woke up one morning and decided to go jogging around the block. Not quite. I went to bed the previous night with a lot on my mind. One of the recurring topics on my spirit was how I wanted to be the person I always imagined myself to be. I was done with settling for less than I deserved. I knew that my life's calling was bigger than my waist size. I wanted to become one of the successful people I admired and respected in the world. In order to do that, I needed to commit to change. I read somewhere that successful people get up early and exercise. They don't wait for sunlight or alarm clocks to control their day. Instead they set their intentions and actions into completing the task of the day.

I'd pull myself out of bed and drink a glass of water. The water would replace my need to fill my stomach up with food. I replaced the processed foods in my home with fresh fruit and veggies. I learned to implement cooking healthier into my daily routine. Even though I would get up early I struggled with my mindset. My mind told me over and over again I was crazy for stepping outside my routine. My body would ache all over the more I tried to move it. I wanted to rest comfortably on my couch and watch tv for hours. Change comes with the conditioning of the mind. I needed to reinforce positive thoughts into my subconscious. Instead of talking myself back into old habits, I learned to speak positively into myself daily. I would leave notes on my nightstand, dresser, bathroom mirror, and television to remind me that I was moving in the right direction. Instead of sitting still for hours, I created a habit of loving to move my body. My body started to really feel like it belonged to me instead of a stranger. Once I was able to alter my morning routine, my life changed for the better. I didn't see the day ahead filled with annoying tasks and ways to escape my reality with food. For the first time in my adult life, I learned to really appreciate the beauty of starting my day on the right foot.

We often become complacent in our daily routines. We get stuck in our comfort and blinded by our negative thoughts. You have the power to take control over your life. The same way we pick up the poor eating habits throughout our lives, we can break them. We have the power of choice. It takes twenty one days to create a new habit. Most people fail because they put so much pressure on themselves to get it right the first day. They often burnout by day two. Understand that creating the bad habits did not happen overnight. You picked them up from your family, friends, and society. The moment you decide to take a step in the right direction to create a new healthy habit, you begin to challenge the cycle of bad habits. All you have to do is start and take it one day at a time. I suggest starting in the morning. It does something to your spirit to see the sunrise and greet the new you.

11

Change Your Mind and You Change Your World

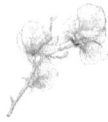

Let's talk about our minds for a sec. When you think of your mind, what do you associate your mind with? Some people look at their mind as a sponge that absorbs information constantly. Others refer to their minds as muscles that need to be sharpened constantly throughout our lifetimes. My mind was a metaphoric construct in which I disappeared when food let me down emotionally and spiritually. I remember those days when I would eat something just to be eating it. My mind told me that I wanted this particular thing and I ran with the idea. I needed to satisfy that part of my mental department to fulfill the missing pieces inside of me. I'd stuff my face until my jaws grew tired. At some point, it wasn't about the satisfaction of the taste. I was controlled by my mind.

My mind was weak when it came to food. This was my fault. I'd conditioned myself to believing that food would always be the answer to my problems in my life. If something was bothering me internally, whether in the workplace or personal relationships, I couldn't verbalize my emotions. I didn't have those sacred relationships in my life that allowed me a safe space to be vulnerable. When life became too much for me to handle, I decided to eat my way through my problems. Nothing was ever quite enough to fill the depth of the void growing inside of me. I'd get down to the last crumb in a bag of chips and feel immense regret. Regret for not having good eating habits. Regret for the way my body became a walking billboard for a health crisis. I eventually had to come to the conclusion that not only was my body sick, so was the state of my mind.

Like so many people struggling with their weight today, I wanted to get better. I used to imagine what I would look like as a size 6. I'd think about all the women who battled with food addiction and how they would one day come up to me and ask for advice on weight loss. They would look at me with hope in their eyes because I could relate to their struggle with food. I wanted to be one of those infomercial models who held their size 16 up to their before and after picture. I had it all figured out in my head about how much better my life would be once I lost the weight. However, my reality and my dream were further apart than I liked to admit.

The idea of going to the gym and watching people stare at me held me captive. I didn't want all those eyes on me. I didn't want anyone's pity over my weight issue. Other people's opinions and judgement would cripple me into body shaming myself. Even if people never said anything like that, I knew in my mind what they were indeed thinking. I'd grown comfortable on my couch and I hid from myself inside my home. I didn't want to look at my changing body in the mirror. I hated the fact that my thighs rubbed together as I walked. I hated the fact that throughout the day all I could think about was the food I was going to eat when I get home. I was beginning to loathe my existence. I was self-destructing and no one could save me.

That is, until my grandmother came to me in a dream. I remember sitting at my grandmother's table as a little girl. She was in the kitchen humming and flipping her wrist. The kitchen smelled of apple pies and cinnamon. It was as if I was watching a movie through my younger self's eyes. My feet could barely touch the floor. But I remember vividly sitting at my grandmother's table with pigtails in my hair and a floral print dress. I sat there waiting for my grandmother, with her peppered hair, to turn towards me and smile. She never looked at me. Instead she dipped her hand in the batter inside the bowl and told me to sit still for a while. I did as I was told and folded my hands inside my lap. The sound of my grandmother's voice caused chills to go down my spine. I wanted so desperately to wrap my arms around her waist and bury myself in her bosom. Something stopped me from moving or speaking in her presence. Her words bounced off my ears as she began to speak. I could remember feeling restless in my spirit. My body felt heavy and my heart began to ache in pain.

"Wipe your tears. Big girls don't cry in this family."

My grandmother warned me. I wiped my eyes and listened closely. In her stern voice, my grandmother told me she'd been watching over me since the day she left this earth. She wasn't too pleased with the way I'd been carrying myself in this world. The little girl in me wanted to explain that I was just going through something.

"Nonsense." My grandmother replied. "You stuck on your tail and need to look within yourself to change your life. You got all the excuses in the world. You just need one solution to change your life."

Her words hit me like a ton of bricks. I remember feeling the tears fall down my cheeks on to my pillow. I could feel my soul begin to open up to my grandmother's words and truth. She didn't raise me to give up on the first, second, or third try in life. She taught me how to be resilient in the face of adversity. Even when I felt like there was nothing left to give, I needed to search for the parts of me that still believed. Even though I couldn't touch my grandmother in my dream, I knew I wasn't the same woman I was the night before. I realized that it was time for me to stop hiding from the world and myself. I realized that the changes I was looking to make in my life would begin with me and the conditioning of my mind.

I didn't need a miracle pill to absorb all of my calories. I didn't need a trainer screaming at me about moving my body. I needed to learn to build a foundation of love, hope, and trust of self within my mind. My mind was under spiritual warfare. I was taking the way I felt about myself internally out on myself externally. Everything that I loved about myself I hid from the world because my mind had convinced me I wasn't worthy. My journey of unlearning everything that I thought I knew and loved about myself was a battle within me. It was not easy learning to change my mind and reinforce positive thoughts and habits. Instead of feeling sorry for myself about my pants size. I conditioned my mind to believe that the number on my pants size was not final. I was in control of my life. I was making changes that I would see externally.

The journey of becoming the woman I always imagined didn't happen overnight. It didn't happen in a few days or weeks. The change began to occur in my life after months of hard work, dedication, and consistency. The most challenging and uncomfortable part was getting used to strengthening my mental health. Most people look for the rewards and benefits of their new habits in their physical appearance. My body was definitely changing. But the way I talked to myself through the good times and bad was proof enough for me. If you can change your mind you can change your life.

You are not stuck inside your body. You are bigger than the number on a scale. You are not the calories you consume on a daily basis. You are not other people's perceptions or ideals of weight loss. You are a work in progress and there is no shame in that. You have the will power and ability to change your life the moment you decide to do so. We often compare our stories to those on television screens or magazine co-vers. I can tell you that half of what you see is makeup and smoke. Just because the body is healthy on the outside doesn't mean the mind is healthy internally.

To change your mind, you have to begin changing the way you speak to yourself. Don't come down on yourself for having ice cream. Instead tell yourself that you only need to have ice cream in moderation. Begin to implement more fruits and veggies into your diet. Get active in your community. When you begin to love and appreciate yourself, you begin to make your mind stronger and sharper. Turn off the television and pick up a book that will plant positive seeds inside of you. Trust me, you're going to need them for your transformation. You owe it to yourself to become the best you possible in this life. Nothing will ever change if you constantly tell yourself that where you are today is your final destination. The cycle ends when you decide that enough is enough and you're going to do something about it.

12

Be Grateful for Failures

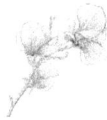

"Think like a queen. A queen is not afraid to fail.
Failure is another stepping stone to greatness."
-Oprah

When I decided to change my life, I knew failure was a part of the equation. I had one thing on my mind − making sure that my life was a success story for people to tell for years to come. Coming from the bottom meant that I would have to continually prove myself in different rooms. For a long time, that bothered me. I wore my heart on my sleeve and believed that everyone was conspiring to see me fail. I can remember there were times where I didn't feel like showing up for work or completing a project. Despite how brilliant my ideas would be or how much I proved my loyalty to the organization, it was never enough. Everything would emotionally drain my spirit and leave me feeling empty on the inside. I didn't consider myself valuable enough to be in the room with people who were way more accomplished than me. Even during those times when I showed up with a bright smile and a receptive spirit, something would always remind me that no matter how far I went in life I would always have to prove myself time and time again.

It was one thing for me to be a woman with ambitions and ideas. It was a different ballpark for me as a woman of color. Men felt threatened by my intelligence. Other women felt intimidated by my intelligence and would sabotage my work. Each time I felt confident about taking a step forward, I was shoved backward ten steps. I knew I would be battling failure my entire journey. Failure? What exactly does that look like? Many people would consider failure not finishing high school or working a dead-end job for minimum wage, though failure may be defined differently for everyone. To me, failure was convincing myself that I didn't deserve to move forward in life. That everyone was essentially right about me being a small-town poor black girl. In my mind, failure equated to a downward spiral of pulling my weight upward in society. I'd occupy spaces I was not invited into or make other people uncomfortable. I constantly told myself that I just needed to continue to show up, even in spaces I was not expected. At times, I'd grow so uncomfortable that I would shrink myself down to nothing. I'd leave in regret for not putting myself forward. The truth of the matter is the odds were against me. I was doomed to fail no matter how hard I tried.

That is, until I remembered how Oprah started her career as a newscaster. She reported the news. She showed up for work and looked for her place in conversations that her name was not mentioned in yet. Even though she failed multiple times as a woman of color in media, her perseverance and tenacity paid off. I could personally and professionally relate to Oprah's public struggles with her weight. People could never completely understand the weight of pressure someone like Oprah or myself would be under to meet and exceed expectations. If I learned anything from Oprah, it is that failure is not an option when you have the faith of a mustard seed. That mustard seed may look like it is just an ordinary seed on the outside. But, when it is planted, watered, and nurtured properly, it can sprout up to make a big difference.

My faith was always a part of my DNA. It was the bridge I often took to get to where I was going in this life. Although things often got shaky underneath, I knew my faith would get me through to the end. My mustard seed had been planted in me long before I discovered what my purpose would be in this world. I made it through some of the worst obstacles in my lifetime. I was living proof that failure was not who I am, it was a figment of my imagination.

Try as we might to blame the world for our circumstances and challenges, we have the power to overcome any obstacle in our path. Life will always hand us a predicament that will make us question if we have the willpower to withstand the test. Trust me, you do. You're not a failure because you have fallen short of your own expectations. You're not a failure if you have to start over or take a different route to the destination. Failure is only possible when you completely choose to give up on everything you believe in. Why would you ever give up when you fight so hard to live each day? It does not make sense to turn your back on your future when you are so close to your breakthrough moment. You owe your future self the ability to see everything you've prayed for manifested in your life.

Sometimes we shrink and disappear within ourselves because that's where we are comfortable. Being comfortable will get you nowhere in life. Everything that you want will be on the other side of your comfort zone. Everyone wants to have a success story that they can pass along to their children — a motivator for their children and grandchildren to pursue a life they will absolutely love. If you give up now and enter failure, you won't have a success story to tell your children.

We often look at successful people in our society as geniuses or experts. We want to know their secret formula for being mega rich, powerful, and influential to others. Successful people are successful because they continuously put one foot in front of the other. They have businesses, ideas, and even partnerships that go south. But, instead of dwelling on what went wrong or who's to blame for the mistakes, they choose to go back to the drawing board and strategize. You are a success from the moment you start to push forward. Don't worry about the results or what other people will think of you in the process. Those who are watching from the sideline are wishing they were as bold and courageous as you.

13

Stop the Guilt, Focus on Yourself

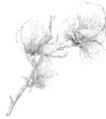

E ven if you do all the right things guilt is an inevitable obstacle on the road to self-improvement. Before I took a deep look inside and decided to dedicate the time to work on myself, feelings of worthlessness hung over my head like a dark cloud. I felt controlled by worthlessness, like a puppet whose every movement and action was dictated by the hands of a sense of self-deprecation and hatred that prevented me from loving myself and blossoming into the strong person I am today. When all you know is a world of devastating worthlessness, the decision to work on yourself is bound to lead to feelings of guilt.

I never felt like I was enough. Whether it was in my personal relationships or professional pursuits, I always felt like the world was trying to bring me down and bury me beneath its soil of self-loathing. When all you can do is hate yourself, working towards self-love can often make you hate yourself even more. But you have to remember that you're worth it; the investment of time and energy that you're putting towards the betterment of your mind, body, and soul will pay off − not just in the weight that you lose, but in the spiritual strength that you gain.

Transformation is something you deserve, and there is absolutely no reason to feel any guilt. You have to stop the guilt and focus on yourself. When we feel like we don't deserve something, we feel guilty when we reach out our hands and try to grab it. Guilt should be the last thing on your mind. You have to know that you're worth the dedication and time. It doesn't mean that you're selfish. All it means is that you're doing what's right − you're doing what you need to do to bloom and become beautiful both inside and out. Self-improvement is not selfish. In fact, it's far from it. Working towards becoming the person you want to be is going to help you give so much to the world. Confidently and lovingly giving to yourself allows you to give to others, and that's such a huge part of a healthy mind and body. If we want to live the lives we need to thrive and be our best, it is paramount that we maintain healthy relationships with others. In order to do that, we have to focus on ourselves first.

I wouldn't be here today teaching you how to give yourself strength if I didn't focus on myself first. Feeling guilty was not an option; and I had to learn that in order to be strong so that I could be there for my friends, family, and for you. My goal was to lose weight so that I could be a better person in every respect, and working on being a better person meant putting myself first. That doesn't mean that I never gave any time to a struggling friend or family member; it just means I had to realize that giving myself the time to grow was ok.

If I didn't focus on myself, I would have been so caught up in the idea of perfection that I would never have been able to rise above the feelings of worthlessness that my husband had so harshly instilled in me. For a while, I only focused on spending time and energy to make my toxic marriage work by trying to meet the standards of perfection that my husband made me feel I could never meet. Instead of giving to myself, I only gave to him, further fueling my food addiction and crushing my self-esteem. In order to lose weight and connect with my inner-beauty, I had to focus on making myself better and not the world around me. Losing weight is all about *self-worth*. As you can see, the key word is self. Putting my efforts into working on myself without feelings of guilt helped me to reach the level of success that I always wanted. Focusing on myself helped to get off that couch that I perceived to be so comfy. I had to break out of my comfort zone, which was in fact a zone of self-loathing and unnecessary suffering. Breaking out of my comfort zone meant doing what I needed to do for myself without feeling the guilt surrounding my suffocating need to please others.

Once I realized that developing my own strength was more important than tirelessly working to please others, I was able to build a strong sense of self and fight my food addiction. I gained power from focusing on myself guilt-free because I knew that's what I needed in order to be the best person I could be. I was able to shed weight, love myself, and help others. I had to focus on myself first, or I would not be able to focus time and energy now on helping you realize how beautiful you are. Trust me when I say that you are worth it, and that it's ok to put yourself before others when you're building a better you.

14

Celebrate Your Wins

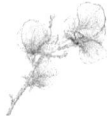

Gaining the strength to lose the weight that's crushing your mind, body, and spirit is undoubtedly something to be celebrated. It's the goal you've been striving toward. So a victory lap is well-deserved. But let's not forget that I said weight loss, and a steady diet of healthy self-affirmation and tough spiritual work, is a constant process that never ends. That shouldn't leave you feeling intimidated. In fact, you should think of it as an opportunity to celebrate more than ever before.

Let's work backward here for a moment and you'll see what I mean. The beginning of kicking my food addiction meant removing sugar from my diet. That sweet tea was such a staple and it seemed that it would be impossible to find anything else to quench my thirst. Of course, I switched to water. A decision to drink water seems pretty simple, but it isn't. That took will power. It isn't just the fact that sweet tea hit the spot in terms of my palette. It was that sweet tea was a means of coping with all the torturous feelings that ruined my self-esteem, causing my self-esteem to drop to even lower depths. Pouring sweet tea down the drain was a win, and a win is always cause for celebration. Now, while taking sweet tea out of the equation wasn't the biggest win of them all, it was certainly a step that deserved recognition. We recognize all milestones in our lives, whether big or small. The refusal to let myself drown in the sea of sweet tea was worth, and still is worth, the celebration. It was a milestone that was key to my success — to both my weight loss and my spiritual gain.

Whatever goal is first on your list, whatever your initial step on your weight loss journey is, you should absolutely celebrate it once you've conquered it. The same goes for the next step, the next one, and so on. Let's not forget that each step is going to vary in terms of the kind of leap that you make. Each step forward is more or less twofold. You're changing your dietary habits, and each change results in a spiritual metamorphosis. Getting off the couch means more than just slimming down your figure; it means changing the way you live your life by changing your mindset.

Go ahead and celebrate checking off a dietary change from your list. It's perfectly reasonable and completely worthy of celebration and praise. But there's no better feeling than reaching a higher spiritual plane − further strengthening the bond between mind, body, and spirit. When you tighten those links, you've reached an unprecedented milestone. I say that because when I realized that every move forward was a holistic one, I felt a fulfilment that I never knew I was capable of feeling.

Major life changes are always worthy of celebrations. Think about graduations, new jobs, marriages, children, therapeutic breakthroughs, overcoming adversity. There's so much potential for us to reach higher and transcend that we often don't realize how much of life is worthy of celebration. All the changes in your diet which lead to changes in your mindset deserve recognition. But remember, maintaining spiritual and emotional success is a process; it isn't a single point that you reach and never have to work towards reaching again. Just think about it. You're going to have so many changes throughout your life, which means there's always going to be more spiritual work to be done – there's going to be more spiritual evolution every time a major life change occurs.

For me, when I had to leave my husband, I was absolutely terrified. Even though he treated me with the highest amount of disrespect imaginable, I still was not comfortable when it all ended. Being married to him for ten years was all that I knew. While I felt liberated, I still had to deal with fear of loneliness and fear of being without a partner. But I overcame that fear, and overcoming it deserved a celebration. I had to deal with a major life change. Once I accepted it and did the work I needed to move on, I knew a celebration was in order. I had won. I had not only defeated the sense of worthlessness that was caused by my husband, but I defeated the initial fear that followed my divorce.

It may seem strange, but the changes that force you to gain your bearings are opportunities for victory and celebration. Let's say that you're laid off for reasons beyond your control. That's a terrifying situation, no doubt. But because you're equipped with the spiritual and emotional strength you developed along your weight loss journey, you'll be completely prepared to deal with the professional change. You have to realize that if you've successfully conquered the negative thoughts that accompany what seem like setbacks, that you'll be able to do anything you want. If you've already overcome the fear associated with losing a job, then great. That means you can overcome the negative thinking that perpetuates your food addiction. You can do anything you want. I promise. I know because the adversity that I conquered seemed absolutely insurmountable until I jumped over the hurdle. My mother left my family, my father was in and out of my life, and I was split apart from my brothers and sisters once we had to enter the foster care system. But then I succeeded in school. I had people tell me I could accomplish anything I wanted. I believed them, and it turns out they were right. I went to college, I received multiple degrees, and I became a therapist which allowed me to live a life that I love. I get to help you do all the things I thought that I couldn't, and nothing brings me greater joy.

If I can do it, then you can do it too. We're all capable of achieving our dreams and every time we meet a goal; we should celebrate our beauty – celebrate the strength we've worked so hard to build. Know that every time you take a step forward, you're reaching a milestone. Celebrate those milestones. It's more than okay to be happy for yourself. Just like any major milestone, you deserve the celebration. You earned it.

15

Creating a Plan for Success

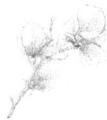

I f you haven't realized it by now, you should know that getting off that couch and transforming the way you live is totally within your grasp. You have more than just the potential to change, meaning this isn't a matter of mere possibility; it's a matter of inevitability. You're absolutely capable of doing everything necessary to lose weight and gain a new perspective, and I'm positive that you'll get everything you want and more. That is a promise.

But I'll make you one more promise: I promise you that your success is dependent upon the hard work that you put into ensuring its fruition. Success doesn't just magically appear overnight. You have to do more than just envision it, than just dream about it. You have to put success into action, and that means you have to make a thorough plan and devise a regimen that's going to fit your unique needs. You have to plan for success because it doesn't just show up at your front door. Before you even map out a plan, you have to make the firm decision to commit to spiritual transformation. You have to look deep within yourself, directly at all that makes you suffer, and you have to take a stand – put your foot down. Say to yourself, it's time to make a change.

You have to not only tell yourself, but you have to *believe* yourself when you say that the time is right to do things differently. You will no longer sit on that couch and watch the beautiful life you know you can live just pass by you while you wonder what could have been. To create a plan, it's crucial that you know in your heart that you're ready to follow a plan. Plans only work if you have the determination to carry them out, and it's you who decides whether you're determined to make the changes or not. I'm here to guide you and motivate you, to encourage you and act as a light when you feel you're just groping in the dark. But even though I'm here for you, that doesn't mean I can make the decision for you as to when you're ready to actually get off the couch. Success only comes when you're ready to welcome it. But you have to consider what welcoming success actually means. Being ready to welcome success means fully understanding the tough road on which you're about to embark; it means accepting that hardship, confusion, second thoughts, doubt, and the desire to give up may very well await you. But you have to remember that those painful feelings are not going to be the end result. They are simply tumultuous steps on the path toward empowerment. I wish I could tell you that it was going to be easy, that this process is going to be a breeze. But lying to you or sugarcoating this would only be doing you a disservice. We already know that pain provides growth, and creating your plan means you have to prepare for that when you decide to take control of your life and lose weight.

Once you fully understand and accept that transformation isn't easy to reach, that you can't just flip a switch and change, then you're ready to create a blueprint for a new inner home that no longer welcomes or hosts negative thinking and self-hatred —a home built on the foundation of determination, strength, and self-empowerment. When creating a plan, you need to begin by figuring out what works for you. Not everyone is going to be able to kick that sugar habit at the same time or slowly phase out certain foods from their diet. Remembering that false perceptions of perfection is a key step here. This is your journey, and you have to understand that if you don't go at your own pace, success will be more difficult to achieve. I've already told you that it's going to be tough, but you'll only make it tougher if you try to swing for the fences right out of the gate. You're a unique individual and that's why you have to create a plan that works for your unique needs. You can't judge your success or create a step by step plan that mirrors the exact path of success as others. When I tell you what worked for me, I'm merely giving you a set of guidelines and showing you that you aren't alone. I know that sharing my journey with you can bring you success. But if I told you that your success should unfold in exactly the same way, I'd be going against much of what I've shared with you.

A huge part of creating a plan means really thinking through the pace at which you can handle changing your habits and adopting a healthy lifestyle. That doesn't mean that you can't handle it. You can handle it. I know it and you know it. But if you try too hard to change right away or if you compare the exact route of your weight loss journey to others, then you could very well fall into the same traps of negative thinking that brought you here in the first place. To set yourself up for success you first have to begin with knowing that you're going to encounter times when you feel like giving up. But it's when you feel like giving up that you know you're doing it right. Understanding that you have to work for success is key to obtaining to it. If you really feel like success should come with the snap of a finger, then you may not be ready to take on the challenge to transform into a new you. I don't say that to put you down; I only mean that you have to plan for a time when you feel like abandoning your plan altogether. When creating a plan — considering pace, particular phases, benchmarks, and checkpoints — you should also remember that you might have to deviate from your plan at certain times. Deviation isn't the same as abandoning the plan, but you have to learn how to adapt quickly to any unforeseen circumstances that might alter the course of your path.

In a way, being unprepared for any curveballs is the same thing as just expecting success to appear without putting in the work. As much as we'd like to think that plans just run smoothly simply because they're laid out, we all know that plans can often change last minute. The type of changes I'm talking about are external factors that many times are out of your control. A big one here is toxic people and rocky relationships — other people who get in the way of your success whether they intend to or not. Take the disintegration of my marriage for instance. Say you're in a similar situation where your husband is cheating on you. No one is really ever totally prepared to handle something like that with calm indifference. It's a heartbreaking situation, and it hurts. If food is your typical coping method and something of that magnitude happens, you may feel like you have no choice but to get back on the couch, sink into the suffocating cushions, and drown yourself in unhealthy foods. You may not even think twice about doing it. Impulsive behavior is such a huge part of addiction, that when you turn to a negative coping mechanism you don't even realize it. If your plans are thwarted because of emotional heartache, the decision can happen in the blink of an eye; almost as if it doesn't seem like a decision at all but more of an automatic reflex.

I'm not saying you should make a separate plan specifically for dealing with a cheating husband, but you might want to at least make a plan for what to do when you're thrown into turbulent circumstances that cause crushing pain and leave you feeling like food is the only way to overcome what seems insurmountable.

Remember that losing weight isn't the only end goal. I've said it time and time again that this all about spiritual balance and wellbeing. Yes, I know you want to bring down your weight and eat healthy; I want that for you as well. But what I really want for you is a healthy spirit; that's what we're trying to obtain here. That's why your plan for success has to be more than just what foods you're going to phase out and when. You have to plan for the emotional aspect of your journey in addition to the surface level component of a new diet (that's not to say building healthy eating habits isn't a difficult thing to do).

When you're putting your plan together, you should write down ways that you'll deal with any sort of circumstance that may trigger you to turn back to the couch. Maybe you find mindfulness exercises to be helpful, or some sort of meditative practice. Maybe you have certain friends or family members you know you can always count on in times of duress (while people can be toxic sometimes, they can also be there to lend a helping hand). Do you find inspiration in books? Do you find prayer helpful? If there's anything out there that you find the slightest bit of inspiration or comfort in, you have to realize that turning to that source is going to be so much better for you than eating your problems away. That's a huge part of what we're doing here, figuring out a new way for you to confront issues and circumstances that cause you unbearable pain. Let's not forget that even though eating is a way you're used to dealing with pain, it only causes more pain. We all know that food addiction – or any addiction – is a vicious cycle. You need to develop new coping mechanisms. Developing those new coping strategies needs to be part of the plan; it's pretty much the crux of your path to success. Working on your diet alone is only solving part of the problem. This transformation is a holistic one. If you don't figure out what you're going to do when the going gets tough, overcoming your food addiction is going to be so much harder to accomplish.

You should also make a plan for sustaining your success once you reach your desired weight. Know that even after you lose weight, you should be planning for how to keep that weight off. By this I don't mean that you should be obsessing about your weight once you shed those pounds. What I'm getting at here is that you should develop a plan for how you deal with anything life throws at you so that you don't fall into the same unhealthy patterns.

When you're embarking on the journey to lose weight, you're ultimately taking a spiritual journey that leads you to the power within you to take control and make the changes you need to flourish in the way you deserve. You know by now that making a deep connection with your inner self and changing the way you think is how you change the way you eat. That means you aren't just making a plan for how to lose the weight; it means you're making a plan that ensures you're always the person you want to be − the type of person who can come out victorious when battling negative thinking. When you look at all the triggers that could potentially thwart your plans to lose weight, think of ways that you can overcome those triggers once you get to where you want to be. Again, this isn't about reaching a certain point. I know that the number on a scale serves as the definite sign of a goal, but that's only one goal that serves to fulfill an ultimate goal. You should absolutely be proud of yourself once you lose weight, but you want to make sure you know how to hold onto that pride. That means you have to plan for your future mindset. We're not trying to achieve temporary solutions here. When making your plan, contemplate how you are going to make sure that you are always the person you want to be.

You have to take so much into account when you think about how you're going to achieve your goals. But I don't want that fact to be a daunting one; I'm not trying to scare you. I want to give you strength and confidence. I'm trying to help you write your guidebook to spiritual change. I don't want you to get lost. Trust me when I say that if you don't make plans for what to do once you reach your goal, then you won't know where to start.

16

Recipes, Meal Plans, and Strategies

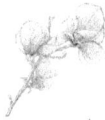

First of all, I want to thank you for letting me be there for you and allowing me into your life to help you reach your weight loss goals. It's truly an honor that you're open to hearing my story. I hope that it inspires you to transform into the most beautiful you just waiting to blossom and bloom for the whole world to see.

Now that you've heard my story and you know what it takes to begin your journey, let's take a look at some tasty recipes that will help you lose weight so you can gain the confidence you want.

Smoothies

I don't know about you, but I absolutely love smoothies. They're a great way to get all the well-rounded nutrients you need all in one in one place, they're easy to prepare, and they taste great. You can also have them on the go so that you can fit healthy living into your busy lifestyle.

Here are some recipes for a handful of my favorites.

BERRY SMOOTHIE

- 1½ cups dairy-free milk
- ½ cup blueberries
- ½ avocado
- 1 cup kale, chopped
- 1 scoop protein powder
- dash of cinnamon

HEALTH SMOOTHIE

- 1½ cups dairy-free milk
- ½ cup pineapple
- 1 cup spinach
- ½ avocado
- 1 scoop protein powder
- dash of cayenne powder

APPLE SMOOTHIE

- 1½ cups dairy-free milk
- 1 apple, chopped
- 1 cup kale, chopped
- ½ avocado
- ¼ inch fresh ginger
- 1 scoop protein powder
- dash of cinnamon powder

GRAPEFRUIT SMOOTHIE

- 1½ cups dairy-free milk
- ½ grapefruit, peeled and chopped
- ½ avocado
- 1 cup spinach
- 1 scoop protein powder
- dash of cayenne powder

FAT BUSTING SMOOTHIE

- 1½ dairy-free milk
- ½ cup blueberries
- ½ avocado
- 1 cup kale, chopped
- 2 tablespoons lemon juice
- 1 scoop protein powder
- 1-inch fresh ginger

For each recipe, you'll want to put all the ingredients in a high-powered blender and mix for 30 seconds. See how easy that was?

Healthy Meal Options

Now let's move on to full meals. As great as smoothies are, you've got to have more than that to maintain a healthy diet, and of course that includes eating nutritional meals. Here are a few of my favorite breakfast options, and one of my favorite dinner options.

Breakfast Options

EGGS WITH AVOCADO AND EZEKIEL TOAST

- – Serves 1
- – 1 tablespoon coconut oil
- – 2 eggs
- – 1 slice Ezekiel bread, toasted
- – 1 avocado, sliced
- – sea salt and black pepper to taste

SCRAMBLE EGGS. Add coconut oil to a medium-sized pan over medium heat. While the oil is melting, crack two eggs into a small bowl and whisk. Pour the eggs into the pan and use a spatula to scramble until firm. Serve the eggs on toast. Top with sliced avocado, sea salt, and black pepper.

BREAKFAST SCRAMBLE WITH SPINACH AND GOAT CHEESE

- Serves 1
- 1 tablespoon coconut oil
- 3 eggs
- 2 cups baby spinach
- sea salt and black pepper to taste
- 1-ounce goat cheese

COOK OMELETTE. Add coconut oil to a medium-sized pan over medium heat. As the oil is melting, crack the eggs in a small bowl and whisk until smooth. Next, add spinach to the pan and sauté until wilted. Season with sea salt and black pepper. Add whisked eggs and use a spatula to scramble. About halfway until the eggs are firm, add goat cheese. Allow the heat to firm up the eggs and serve.

SUPER VEGGIE SCRAMBLER

- 1 red bell pepper, chopped
- 1/2 medium yellow onion, diced
- 1 medium zucchini, cut into half moons
- 4 oz (half box) mushrooms, sliced
- 2–3 cloves garlic, minced
- 1 Tbsp extra virgin olive oil, butter, vegan spread
- 1-3 Tbsp Organic Coconut Aminos
- Sea salt & pepper, to taste

Prep all the vegetables the night before, or in the morning if you have time. Heat the oil in a large skillet over medium heat. Toss all the veggies in the skillet together (including the garlic and pepper), mix well and cook, stirring every now and then until starting to brown, about 10 minutes. Remove the pan from the heat and serve immediately. Season to taste with salt and freshly milled pepper.

Dinner Option

CAULIFLOWER FRIED RICE

- – 1 head cauliflower should make 4 cups rice
- – 1 teaspoon coconut or avocado oil
- – 1/2 yellow onion *finely diced*
- – 1/2 cup frozen peas/carrots
- – 1/4 teaspoon ground ginger
- – 1 teaspoon red pepper flakes omit if you don't want it spicy
- – 2 large cloves garlic *pressed or minced*
- – 2 tablespoons Organic Coconut Aminos
- – 1/2 - 1 tablespoon lime juice
- – 1/2 cup sliced mushrooms
- – 1 cup spinach

Heat oil over medium heat. Once hot, book onions, carrots/peas, and spices for about 5 minutes or until veggies are soft. Add garlic in the last 30 seconds. Lower heat to medium low. Add cauliflower "rice" and cook about 5 minutes or until desired texture is reached. Stir in coconut Aminos, lime juice, and spinach. Taste and re-season if necessary. Serve as is or with a fried egg, chicken, shrimp, etc.

3 Day Sugar Detox Meal Plan

Remember when I told you about sugar withdrawals? Well, they're the real deal. I was crazy addicted to sugar. When you're kicking an addiction, you need a detox plan. It's just like with drugs. Your body's going to crave what it's addicted to, and those cravings are going to affect your mind and its decision-making process. It's going to take 3 days, but fortunately there's a meal plan you can follow to overcome the withdrawals.

At first it may seem like kicking sugar is going to be the longest 3 days of your life, but trust me when I say this plan is going to make things easier. The foods you eat along the way taste great too! Here's the meal plan you need to stick to in order to get you through that initial rough patch.

DAY ONE

- **Breakfast**: Health smoothie
- **Mid-morning snack**: Nuts
- **Lunch**: Grilled Chicken Breast with mixed baby greens and half an avocado
- **Afternoon snack**: Sliced peppers with two tablespoons of spinach hummus

- **Dinner**: Edamame, salmon with stir-fried broccoli and mushrooms

DAY TWO

- **Breakfast**: Three eggs scrambled with sautéed spinach
- **Snack**: Nuts
- **Lunch**: Tuna Niçoise salad
- **Snack**: Sliced peppers with hummus
- **Dinner**: Salmon, sautéed Brussels sprouts and mushrooms with lettuce salad and avocado

DAY THREE

- **Breakfast**: Three-egg omelet with shrimp, sautéed spinach and tarragon
- **Snack**: Nuts
- **Lunch**: Grilled turkey burger with sliced to-matoes, lettuce, and sautéed mushrooms, plus kale chips
- **Snack**: Sliced peppers with hummus
- **Dinner**: Baked cod over and mixed greens

Drinks allowed over the three day period: One cup of unsweetened black coffee per day, unsweetened green and/or herbal tea in unlimited amounts, minimum 64 ounces of water a day

See? That's three days of well-balanced meals and snacks. Everything on the list will give you the needed nutrients to help keep you sharp and stay full. There's plenty of food to eat, and you won't be left starving at the end of the day. And most importantly, you're going to get through those sugar withdrawals while eating healthy.

What's really great about starting the journey with meals such as these, is that your body is going to get used to eating such healthy foods. Not only are these meals a way to get you through the sugar withdrawals, but they'll help you develop healthy eating habits that you'll definitely learn to love.

Strategies for continued success

You already know how important preparation and planning is to losing weight. When considering how to keep your healthy diet consistent, that is also something you're going to have to be prepared for. It's more than just planning for a diet to help you lose weight; it's planning for a diet that's going to help you keep the weight off. You should always have on hand only the foods that are going to keep you trim and happy. When you do your grocery shopping, make sure that you only buy food and ingredients that you need – nothing more. You have no reason to buy food that does not fit into the plan. It would just derail you, and you might end up making meals that won't contribute to your success. It's all about knowing exactly what you need, when you need it.

You want everything that you have on hand to be foods that will ensure continued success. And you definitely only want to have foods arounds that you know you have the time to prepare. Don't get too out of control and overwhelm yourself with meals you might not be able to make or are just too busy to do so.

It's also good to make sure you prepare your snacks ahead of time. If everything is ready come morning, you won't be stressed trying to put together healthy snacks before you run out the door. If you don't have healthy foods on hand, you may be tempted to just grab foods that are unhealthy, or get a quick fatty breakfast at a fast food restaurant.

Make sure you always have lots of leafy greens at home. Not only are they healthy for both your body and mind, but there are so many quick dishes you can make with leafy greens. This is definitely an instance of a little going a long way.

You can quickly sauté spinach with some garlic, olive oil, and salt and pepper. And don't forget how quick it is to make a salad, soup, or a green-based smoothie.

Just making sure to consistently have veggies around is a great idea. Peppers, carrots, beets, asparagus, green beans, celery, and cucumbers can be prepared easily; some of them you can eat raw and snack on during the day. If you're at work, you can pack some of those veggies in a plastic bag to bring with you for a nice mid-morning snack.

And of course, you're going to want to make sure you throw some fruits in your diet. Apples, bananas, berries, and oranges are great quick and easy snacks.

Avocados are great to have around since you can use them to prepare meals and snacks just as quickly. They're great to add to toast, or you can throw them in your salad. They're also a wonderful snack on their own with a little sea salt and pepper, or cumin sprinkled on top. And let's not forget hummus. It's a healthy dip and you can also use it as a salad dressing.

Keeping grass-fed meat around the house is a great idea too, and you can never go wrong with wild fish. Get meats like easy shredded chicken. It cooks quickly and you can cook it in big batches if you want to save some for later. If you're someone who has a sweet-tooth, medjool dates are great to have around for satisfying any cravings for sweet foods.

Of course, making sure you stay active is key. This doesn't mean that you have to hit the gym seven days a week, pump iron, and run on the treadmill. If working out is your thing, then go for it. But for many people (including myself) a workout is kind of boring; but you can't stay stagnant. I incorporate many different activities during my workout to make them fun and exciting. I also enjoy working out with others because it helps to keep me motivated. Just doing little things like going for walks can do wonders. If there's a sport you enjoy, then go outside and play it. Sports are an excellent way to play while keeping your body healthy. If you have a bike, hop on and ride it. You want to make sure you're active while doing things you enjoy. Staying active shouldn't be boring; you don't need to make it feel like it's a chore.

I know that losing weight is likely your goal here, and exercising and staying active to lose weight is a great way to get there and stay there. But an even bigger goal is your happiness and wellbeing. Making a change shouldn't be miserable, even if misery is what sparks you to change.

At this point you probably understand that you have to actively keep your emotional health in check as well. Staying active is more than just moving your body; it's working on the perpetual development of your mind and spirit. Reaching success takes hard work, and you have to always put in the spiritual work to keep it. But of course, you shouldn't think of emotional and mental work as a chore. Yes, often working on your inner self can be hard. It always takes a courageous soul to confront your fears, sadness, and ask what you can do differently to transform the way you think. But you must remember what that work can bring you: happiness, love, serenity, and strength.

Your wellbeing is an investment that is absolutely worth the continual work. This is about building a better life for yourself and maintaining a healthy state of mind to help you live a full life. Working to ensure emotional health is ultimately rewarding, and consistently so. You already know that every victory deserves a celebration, and that every time you overcome pain you grow exponentially. You should never lose sight of the fact that this is all about building an everlasting connection between your mind, body, and spirit. It's about cultivating a strong relationship between you and your inner self.

Losing weight is just a part of building that key connection to a happy and fulfilling life. I'm not saying that losing weight isn't important. I'm only saying that this isn't all about the weight itself. This is all about changing the way you think and feel. Yes, changing the way you think results in changes in your body. But the transformation your body undergoes is more about a transformation of your mind and spirit. Just think of how much empowerment comes from making the choice to lose weight to begin with. You must remember every day that the courage *itself* to lose weight is what brings about your transformation, not just losing the weight. Continued success means realizing what it is that brought you your success, and always keeping the formula for success in mind.

My Thanks to You

Again, I want to thank you so much for allowing me to guide you towards your spiritual transformation. Nothing brings me greater joy than knowing I've helped another woman through struggles that at first seem insurmountable. Though my path was one filled with roadblocks, detours, and great pain, it allowed me to become the person I am and allowed me to help you make changes in your life. I hope that you find inspiration in my story; it's why I've chosen to tell it to you. I truly believe that my struggles were part of a test; a test that once passed, would lead me to a place of strength and spiritual fortitude. If I was not able to pass that test, then I would not be able to help you pass yours. I hope that any shred of inspiration you take away from reading this inspires you to help other women who struggle just like you do and just like I did. That's one of the best things I could ever ask for. It isn't just about inspiring you; it's about inspiring all women to take control of their lives and make a change, to better themselves so that they can do better in the world.

I guarantee you that losing weight and reaching the plane of ultimate spirituality will help you want to give to others. Getting off the couch is about more than you; it's about all women everywhere. Do yourself a favor, do all women a favor. Get off that couch and lose that weight. I want you to truly connect with the beauty inside of you, so that you can feel great about yourself and help other women to do the same. You can get the results if you make yourself a priority. I want to tell you that you are special and awesome and that you have amazing gifts to offer the world! Listen, we are all facing different challenges in life, but I want to encourage you to start changing your mindset. When you change your mindset, you change your life! To start your mindset transformation, I would like you to incorporate affirmations in your daily routine. Affirmations are a great way to help reframe our minds from the negative to positive.

Here are my Daily affirmations that I encourage you to try!

I am LOVED

I am POWERFUL

I am WORTHY

You have the power to change your life today! All you have to do is look deep within yourself and realize your inner strength and infinite potential. You have to believe that you are worthy of the effort required for change. You can achieve success if you just make the effort to get off the couch and change the way you think. I promise. ~Dr. Radisha Brown

BEFORE AFTER

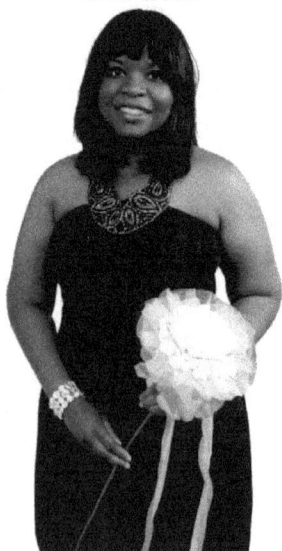 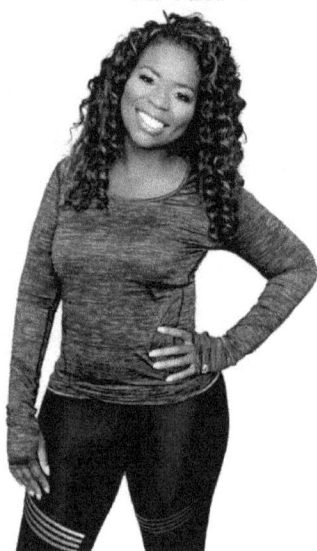

THANK YOU LADIES!

A special **Thanks** to the below list of amazing female entrepreneurs. I affectionately call you my "Inner Circle of Inspiration!" Some I have known for years~ others I have never met but nonetheless, you have all played a part in my journey!

Natalie Bryan
PEARL Inc
www.wearepearl.org

Jasmine Dawson
Jasmine Dawson Marketing
jasminedawson281@gmail.com

Mimi Davis
A La Carte Marketing
www.a-la-carte-marketing.com

Min. Nakita Davis
Jesus Coffee & Prayer
www.jesuscoffeeandprayer.com

Ticora Davis
The Creator's Law Firm
www.creatorslawfirm.com

Dionne Dunn

My Serenity Retreats
www.myserenityretreats.com

Racheal Feldman
Your Health Coach Biz
www.rachelafeldman.com

Kissha Heyward
Mary Kay Consultant
www.marykay.com

Kim Honeycutt
Peer In Counseling Center
www.butyourmotherlovesyou.com

Ericka D James
Kingdom Ministers
www.erickajackson.com

Shanta Johnson
Essential Cleansing Center
www.essentialcleansingcenter.com

Keisha Kells
Perfected Practice
www.perfectedpractice.com

Amy D Kilpatrick
Nspired Business Solutions
www.nspiredbusinesssolution.com

Jessica LeeAnn
Chocolate Readings
www.chocolatereadings.com

Cyndyl McCutcheon
Cyndyl McCutcheon
@cyndyl13

Jennifer Niu
Certified Health Coach
@Jennifer Niu

Heather Parady
Heather Parady
www.HeatherParady.com

Bethany Smith
Bethany Smith Yoga
www.bethanysmithyoga.com

Spirit
T2S Enterprises
www.talk2spirit.com

Samara Stone
The Stone Foundation
www.perfectedpractice.com

MC Walker
Walker Publication
www.themcwalker.com

Nicole Walters
Monetize Thyself
www.nicolewalters.com

Stacy Washington
Xubian Acne Clinic
www.xubianacneclinic.com

Gianna Williams
Stylez By Gianna
@stylezbygianna

Health Book Resources

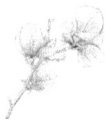

[Paleo Cooking from Elana's Pantry: Gluten-Free, Grain-Free, Dairy-Free Recipes](#)

by [Elana Amsterdam](#)

Eat Dirt: Why Leaky Gut May Be the Root Cause of Your Health Problems and 5 Surprising Steps to Cure It by Josh Axe

A Mind of Your Own: The Truth About Depression and How Women Can Heal Their Bodies to Reclaim Their Lives by Kelly Brogan and Kristin Loberg

The Paleo Approach Cookbook: A Detailed Guide to Heal Your Body and Nourish Your Soul by [Sarah Ballantyne](#)

The Complete Anti-Inflammatory Diet for Beginners: A No-Stress Meal Plan with Easy Recipes

to Heal the Immune System by [Dorothy Calimeris](#) and [Lulu Cook](#)

Wheat Belly: Lose the Wheat, Lose the Weight, and Find Your Path Back to Health by William Davis

Food: What the Heck Should I Eat? by Mark Hyman

Body Love: Live in Balance, Weigh What You Want, and Free Yourself from Food Drama Forever by Kelly LeVeque

The Nutrient-Dense Kitchen: 125 Autoimmune Paleo Recipes for Deep Healing and Vibrant Health 1st Edition by Mickey Trescott

9 780999 818848